Intermittent Fasting For Women

Beat The Food Craving And Get That Weight Shaving

James Brook

The trademarks that are used are without any consent, and the publication of the trademark is without permission or backing by the trademark owner. All trademarks and brands within this book are for clarifying purposes only and are the owned by the owners themselves, not affiliated with this document.

Table Of Contents

Introduction

Well done and congratulations for downloading this book,

"Intermittent Fasting For Women: Beat The Food Craving And Get That Weight Shaving!".

In this book you will find a plethora of valuable information regarding a way of eating that is gaining popularity at a rapid pace in the health and fitness world. This diet protocol, intermittent fasting, comes backed with scientific evidence to support a multitude of health benefits such as weight loss, increased mental alertness, and even a longer lifespan that women all of ages can enjoy.

In a society becoming more and more satisfied with sedentary lifestyles, poor diet choices, and soaring waistlines, there are a growing number of rebels out there fighting this detrimental norm. These individuals realize that our bodies are the most important asset we will ever have, and that we only get one of them! If you are taking the time to read the information in this book, it means that you are probably one of these people, good for you.

For as long as people have been concerned with getting or staying in shape and maintaining a healthy diet, there have always been certain diet plans that explode in popularity, only to fizzle out over time when people decide that they are impractical, unhealthy, or just plain ineffective. There are, however, some diet plans that have stood the test of time, helping individuals achieve their physical goals while providing structure and maintainability.

Intermittent fasting is a diet plan that has been around since the dawn of mankind, only receiving its formal name in recent years. In all honesty, our early ancestors probably adapted this kind of diet out of necessity, as you will understand later, but its benefits are being reaped by many people even today. This book will focus on the ins and outs of intermittent fasting from a woman's perspective, and provide a guideline of how to effectively implement it into your daily life, as well as explain possible hazards and how you can avoid them.

Before we get into this information I would like to answer a question that has been posed countless times, that is "what is the best diet plan to follow"? The answer to this question is simple, the one you will stick to! After completing this book, I hope you will decide that intermittent fasting is right for you, and enjoy the many health benefits and convenience that it provides.

Chapter 1: What Is Intermittent Fasting?

In today's modern food culture, we have been conditioned for the entirety of our lives that we need to eat throughout the day to keep our bodies healthy. You have probably heard over and over that breakfast is the most important meal of the day, or that eating small meals every 2-3 hours is ideal for an efficient metabolism. The truth is, eating with this kind of frequency is not the way our species were made to function, and is actually a relatively new trend amongst the human race.

By giving the body a break, such as following the intermittent fasting lifestyle, we are able to become a healthier, more efficient physical machine that performs at the level it was designed for. So what is Intermittent Fasting? Answering this question is probably a good idea before we discuss any further details about it. Intermittent Fasting, put simply, is a diet protocol in which you do not eat throughout the day, consuming all of your daily calories within a specific eating window that you designate. The time that you spend fasting throughout the day is usually far longer than the eating window.

The key aspect to point out here is that you are not consuming any CALORIES during the fasting period, you are still free to consume as much water as you need (very important), as well as any flavored drinks or dietary supplements that you choose as long as they are calorie free. For example, most people that adhere to intermittent fasting engage in a 16 hour fast day, followed by an 8 hour eating window. One of the benefits of this protocol is that you can decide on your eating window based on your lifestyle, making intermittent fasting very convenient.

If you are an early bird, being most productive early in the day and usually in bed when the sun goes down, you can choose to eat earlier, say from 9am-5pm. For all the night owls out there who see midnight on a regular basis, pushing your eating window back to 4pm-12am is not problem at all. Any way you design your intermittent fasting plan is fine, so long as you follow the foundational rules: no calories during your fasting period (while still staying properly hydrated), and sticking to consuming all of your calories during the strict eating window that you designate.

If this is your first time of hearing intermittent fasting, you may be ready to close it immediately and never even consider this lifestyle. If that is you, this feeling is probably due to outdated fitness and nutrition advice that society and so-called "gurus" have hammered into your mind for decades. You have without a doubt heard that breakfast is the most important meal of the day, or eating 5-6 small meals every 2-3 hours throughout the day is the most effective way for efficient metabolism, or that 'starving' yourself in an attempt to lose weight is counterproductive, etc.

Before we even begin to debunk these myths with all of the benefits of intermittent fasting, you need to realize that this is not a new concept by any means. Eating throughout the course of the entire day is a relatively new concept. Food has become so convenient and accessible in today's society that we are trained into believing we need three square meals a day. Society is so concerned with eating, instant gratification of our dietary desires that there are fast food restaurants on every corner with their flashing neon signs advertising the latest $5 calorie bomb. Is it any surprise then, that obesity levels are soaring, heart disease and stroke are running rampant, and people are more unhealthy than ever before?

From our earliest ancestors all the way up until a few hundred years ago, the habit of eating one large meal at the end the day was the norm. Ancient humans were hunter-gatherers, spending the entire day foraging for edible vegetation, hunting game, and just trying to survive. Eating was considered a celebratory ritual and was accompanied by a feast each evening when the food was brought back to the tribe. Even our modern ancestors spent their days farming the land, working whatever job needed to be done for their families, eating one large meal after a hard day's work.

While I am by no means saying that these people had it better than we do now (I would rather eat a few too many calories each day than have to survive a saber-toothed tiger attack), they did in fact reap many of the benefits of intermittent fasting without even realizing it. To digress, eating throughout the duration of the day is a relatively new concept that is not at all necessary to a healthy lifestyle.

Now that we have discussed the basics of what intermittent fasting is and its place in human history, we will go over some of the many benefits of following this dietary lifestyle.

Chapter 2: What Are The Scientific Benefits Of Intermittent Fasting?

The first and most obvious benefit of intermittent fasting is that by following this protocol, you are far more likely to consume fewer calories during the day. The foundation of any weight loss plan is often lost behind complicated diet plans and flawed philosophies that serve to confuse people more than they help them. This foundation is that calories are the key to weight gain or loss. If you consume fewer calories per day than your body burns, you are going to lose weight. Likewise, if you take in a surplus of calories compared to what your body burns, weight gain is inevitable.

What happens when we eat regular meals all throughout the day? You wake up, eat breakfast, and then usually even before lunch you get hungry again, indulging in a snack here and there. After lunch, we usually have a 4-6 hour wait before dinner and then more snacks to satisfy our urges tend to follow. With this constant cycle of eating, getting full, and then getting hungry again and eating more between meals, it makes it so easy for us to consume too many calories throughout the day. With intermittent fasting, once your body adjusts to the prolonged fasting period, you will eat fewer meals because you are limited to a timed 'feeding' window. This allows you to prevent excess hunger between meals and feel relatively satiated throughout the duration.

For example, the average person is advised to follow a 2,000-calorie per day diet. Which do you think is more difficult to achieve, eating throughout the entire day, 3 meals and snacks included, while only consuming 2,000 calories, or only allowing yourself 8 hours to eat the same number? Obviously it is easier to eat a healthy number of calories if you limit them to a shorter window. Intermittent fasting will allow you to more easily consume your desired number of calories than eating all day will.

Another profound benefit of intermittent fasting is an increase in insulin sensitivity in the body. Insulin is a hormone released into the bloodstream when there is a rise in blood glucose. It serves to regulate, in this case decrease and breakdown, our blood glucose levels and maintain a proper balance. As we discussed earlier, our society is experiencing an obesity epidemic of epic proportions. Hand in hand with obesity is type 2 diabetes. Type 2 diabetes results when the body is unable to use insulin properly. When this happens, the pancreas (the organ that produces insulin) will attempt to produce extra insulin at first, but will eventually be unable to keep up, causing blood glucose levels to soar.

Obesity is associated with type 2 diabetes due to the fact that when the pancreas has to constantly release a large amount of insulin (typical of a poor diet, a primary cause of obesity), eventually the insulin receptors in the body become overloaded and lose their ability to use insulin efficiently. According to the Center for Disease Control and Prevention, almost 90% of the people living with type 2 diabetes are obese or overweight.

The *Journal of Applied Physiology* performed a study on individuals to determine the effects of intermittent fasting on insulin sensitivity. The study selected eight subjects, and had them fast for twenty hours per day, every other day, for a fifteen-day duration. After fifteen days, the subjects' blood was examined and researchers concluded that their glucose uptake levels (the breakdown of glucose characteristic of proper insulin function) was much more efficient than the baseline established before the fasting protocol began.

The study went even further with an explanation as to why they may have seen these results. It is believed that our human genome was finalized sometime around the late Paleolithic era (50,000-10,000 BC). As we discussed earlier, this came at a time when there were no guarantees when it came to finding food each day. Not only did Paleolithic man engage in frequent physical activity in their pursuit for sustenance, but they also experienced regular fluctuations between feast and famine. This fasting lifestyle period early man experienced just so happened to be the period of time our genome was selected, so it makes sense as to why our metabolisms seem to be more efficient with this type of diet.

As we discuss obesity, losing weight, and burning fat, let's use basic human biology to explain why we store fat in the first place. The human body is an incredible machine, it is designed to survive many hardships, and famine is one of them. When we consume an excess of calories, the body will use as many calories as it needs at the time, but then store away the rest as either glycogen in the liver, but more readily, as adipose tissue (or fat).

This was extremely necessary for the ancient man, when food was scarce and unavailable for sometimes days on end; the body used the fat it had stored during times of plentiful food to survive. Fat however, is not the body's go to source for fuel in normal situations. If food is readily available, it will use glucose as a primary energy source, saving the fat for more drastic times. In today's world, with eating all throughout the day as the norm and food more readily available than ever before, the average persons body today tends to get its energy almost exclusively from glucose. We never experience that famine situation in which our fat stores were designed to withstand.

As advanced as we think we've become in our society, it is ironic that our actual genome has changed very little since ancient humans. Even today, if we engage in intermittent fasting, we actually signal to the body that we are experiencing a period of scarce food and, once the body gets used to this protocol, we actually see a shift in its primary energy source. By following the intermittent fasting protocol, we can train the body to start using our fat stores for energy instead of glucose alone. Most overweight people today are caught in a cycle where the blood glucose is always elevated due to being full. When this starts to decrease, instead of their body switching to burning fat as fuel, they simply get hungry and eat again. This not only keeps blood glucose way too high consistently, but also does not allow the body to burn fat like it otherwise would.

Another little known, but monumental, benefit of intermittent fasting is that it has been shown to decrease the odds of contracting breast cancer in women, and also aid in the fight against cancer in general once a woman has developed it. A study of 7,000 women with a history of anorexia actually showed a 50% reduction in the incidence of breast cancer. Before we go any further yes, anorexia is a horrible disease in itself but what researchers took from this was that caloric restriction and fasting, all characteristic of anorexia, decreases breast cancer risks. According to Alex Lickerman, MD, of *Psychology Today*, intermittent fasting has also been shown to reduce the side effects of chemotherapy and even increase its effectiveness when used immediately before and after chemo.

There have been an extensive amount of studies that indicate calorie restriction, is actually indicative of a longer life. The two studies we will focus on took place at the University of Wisconsin-Madison (UWM), and the National Institute on aging (NIA). The study uses rhesus monkeys as the test subjects. These monkeys are a good choice for making conclusions about the human body, as we share a wide variety of anatomical and biological similarities. All of the monkeys in the UWM study that were subjected to caloric restriction, did in fact live longer than the control group.

But ladies, listen to this: the male monkeys lived, on average, two years longer than the control group. The females, however, lived an average of SIX years longer by restricting their calories! Four of the monkeys in the NIA study actually broke longevity records for rhesus monkey age, living as long as forty years when the average lifespan for this species is around thirty years of age. Not only did the monkeys in both of these studies live longer, they also experienced much lower incidents of cancer and heart disease. The two go hand in hand with longevity if you consider the fact that cancer and heart disease are always at the top of the list of death for both men and women.

What an enormous benefit to gain from a change in diet. Literally everything we do with proper nutrition and exercise, goes back to trying to live as long as we can and be healthy while we are here. Intermittent fasting has consistently shown to increase the lifespan of numerous animals, which is what you and I are as well! Not to mention that living a healthy and happy life is one of the most important things to do while we live on this beautiful planet.

Another positive side effect associated with intermittent fasting is improved brain health. I think we can all agree that the brain is a fairly important organ to look out for, as even agreeing with this statement requires the brain. A study by a group of Canadian researchers showed that prolonged periods of fasting in animals actually slowed down the flow of information across the neurons in the brain. Although slowing down our brains may seem counter intuitive, this actually benefits our mental health.

The stress of day-to-day life which we all experience has our neuronal circuits constantly firing, leaving the brain overworked by our tedious schedules. Too much activity in the synapses of the brain, (which are responsible for relaying information) has been linked with several diseases of the brain and nervous system, such as Alzheimer's and Parkinson's disease. It seems as if the slowing down of the brain through fasting gives it a break, allowing it to recharge. When in a fasting state, the body produces compounds known as ketone bodies, which are known to protect the neurons in the brain, preventing them from degrading to the point of disease. Furthermore, intermittent fasting has even been proven extremely effective in combating depression and anxiety.

'Brain-derived neurotrophic factor' is a chemical released in the brain that is responsible for the formation of neuronal networks. In people suffering from depression, we see this chemical suppressed substantially. When these new neuronal networks have a difficult time forming and branching out, depression is far more likely. A study from the *Neurobiology of Disease* in 2007 concluded that periods of fasting can actually increase the concentration of Brain-Derived Neurotrophic factor anywhere from 50 to 400 percent! We're not talking about a slight increase here, this is a huge amount.

Another chemical chain that occurs in the brain during periods of fasting and caloric restriction, involves a hormone called Ghrelin. Ghrelin is known as the hunger hormone because it increases when we are hungry and/or fasting. When it comes to mental health, however, increased Ghrelin is very helpful. Not only has this hormone been linked to elevated mood, but a study published in the *Journal of Molecular Psychiatry* found that it is actually a natural antidepressant and promotes neurogenesis in the brain.

In our world today, chronic depression and anxiety levels are at an all time high, and people report feeling higher levels of anxiety than ever before. Intermittent fasting can be a useful tool to circumvent this trend and help keep your mood uplifted throughout the day. Not only will this lifestyle alter the chemical balance in your brain, allowing you to combat and prevent depression, but the weight-loss and fitness benefits will serve to improve your self-image and confidence, which are both aspects of life that, when negative, cause depression and anxiety. Think of intermittent fasting as a double-edged sword that slices through both obesity and depression.

Intermittent fasting may seem to be a new trend that has emerged in the spotlight recently, as many fad diet plans often do, but rest assured that this is not a recent new way of life. This lifestyle has been around far longer than you and I have been alive, or even our great-great (times 20) grandparents have been around to consider it.

Today's modern food culture has led us to believe that we must not go any more than a few hours without eating, and that our entire day should be based around meals. The science behind intermittent fasting does not agree. Should you choose to give this lifestyle a try, you could reap all of the benefits that we've discussed and more. While skipping meals and engaging in a prolonged period of fasting may go against all your prior beliefs on eating and how food should be consumed, I strongly believe that you will find the benefits worth the try.

"The light of the world will illuminate within you when you fast and purify yourself." -Mahatma Gandhi

Chapter 3: Specific Effects Of Intermittent Fasting On The Female Body And Precautions For Potential Hazards

In the previous two chapters we explained exactly what intermittent fasting is, as well as some of the benefits one can expect to experience while following this dietary lifestyle. While the effects that we discussed are the same for both men and women, this book is about intermittent fasting for women. Therefore, this chapter will focus on effects of intermittent fasting more specific to the female body. Furthermore, while there are a plethora of benefits that women can reap from choosing to fast, there are also some health concerns unique to women that we should discuss, as well as how you can avoid them. After all, if you choose to begin intermittent fasting to live a healthier and fuller life, the last thing you want is to create new health problems in the process!

We have discussed how intermittent fasting can help both men and women lose weight, have more energy, and even lower their risks for many types of diseases. However, there have been numerous studies performed using only women as subjects where intermittent fasting has proven extremely effective at providing these benefits. A study published in the International Journal of Obesity in 2011 selected two groups of women and subjected them to two different methods of fasting, continuous (no food for an entire day) and intermittent. While both groups of women lost weight, the group that adhered to intermittent fasting saw 30% of the women losing anywhere from 5-10% of their body weight, and

34% of these women lost over 10% of their body weight.

What is even more remarkable about these findings is that these women were not instructed to exercise, and made little if any changes in their amount of physical activity during this study! We are not talking about a few pounds here and there, without even taking exercise into consideration, these women were able to lose a remarkable amount of body weight by just trying intermittent fasting. While this study was performed to see how fasting affected weight loss in women, researchers also wanted to see if this lifestyle was really effective in preventing certain diseases. They measured certain risk markers for things such as diabetes, cancer, and cardiovascular disease in these women before the study began, and immediately afterwards. What they found was that after following the intermittent fasting protocol, these risk markers were decreased substantially in all of the women.

Another study published in the *Nutrition Journal* in 2012 aimed to learn what happened to the energy needs in the female body when fasting begins. A group of women were selected to follow an 8-week, calorically restricted intermittent fasting plan. What they found was that the women's bodies actually had a huge reduction in their body's energy needs, between 75-90%! Intermittent fasting makes the female body incredibly more efficient and teaches it to use energy much more effectively. Once again, the human body is an incredible piece of machinery, and is extremely adaptive and knows how to maintain itself at all costs. When it experiences fasting, it will teach itself to run just as well, if not even better on fewer calories, as it plunges into fat reserves to continue functioning optimally.

Now there are a few health concerns specific to the female body that I would like to address when it comes to intermittent fasting. The first of these are drastic hormonal food cravings. We touched on this subject earlier, but there are numerous hormones in the body that regulate and control hunger. These include insulin, leptin, and ghrelin, among many others. Women subjected to extended periods of fasting (as in not eating for an entire day) are susceptible to having these hormones thrown out of whack.

When this happens, the chemical signals in the brain that let you know when you are full and should not eat anymore become turned off, which can cause overeating. A study consisting of female college students at the University of Virginia had the subjects fast for two whole days. What they found was that levels of leptin in these women decreased by as much as 75%! This can severely disrupt feelings of satiety and result in someone consuming entirely too many calories when the fasting period is over. The women in this study also experienced a 50% increase in their cortisol levels. Cortisol is more commonly referred to as the stress hormone.

Cortisol becomes elevated when we are worn out, nervous, afraid, and/or hungry. It can also cause us to crave sugary, fatty foods to try and feed our body a quick burst of highly available energy. The body craves this quick fix in order to deal with whatever short term situation we are in. This is simply another one of the body's survival mechanisms. As a woman, if you are following intermittent fasting to lose weight, the last thing you want is your cortisol level through the roof, begging you to eat that candy bar or drink a soda! So how can you avoid these hormonal cravings causing you to overeat and desire junk food? Well, instead of going on an extended fast such as 24 to 48 hours, if you will simply narrow your food intake into 8-10 hour feeding windows, you can reap the benefits of intermittent fasting while burning fat and increasing your insulin sensitivity without throwing your hunger hormones for a loop.

Another serious side effect of intermittent fasting unique to the female body is a disrupted menstrual cycle and even a decreased ovary size. A study conducted using female rats found that after two weeks of intermittent fasting, the rat's menstrual cycles ceased completely and their ovaries were severely diminished. This is thought to be yet another survival mechanism in the mammalian body, and sort of makes sense if you think about it. If the female body believes that it is starving, and is trying to use as little energy available as efficiently possible, the last thing that needs to be introduced into this equation is a growing fetus that requires an enormous amount of energy to develop.

If a woman's body believes it is having a hard enough time keeping itself alive, Mother Nature will make some changes, such as bringing ovulation to a halt and shrinking the ovaries. This is to ensure that there will be only one human to keep alive for the time being. While this is a remarkable mechanism of survival that probably served our ancient ancestors well, you are not actually starving, and you most likely do not want to have your reproductive system thrown out of balance. So if you begin intermittent fasting and notice changes in your menstrual cycle and ovulation frequency, what can you do? Dr. Amy Shah, an expert of intermittent fasting protocols and their effects on the female anatomy, recommends what she calls crescendo fasting.

What this entails is that women do not actually fast everyday, but select two to three days out of the week, preferably non-consecutive days such as Monday, Wednesday, and Friday, and fast the usual 12-16 hours during these days. On the days you are fasting, this method recommends women only engage in physical exercise such a light yoga, while saving any high intensity workouts for non-fasting days. After following this method for 2-3 weeks, women are encouraged to try and add one more fasting day during the week, and monitor their body's reaction. By partaking in crescendo fasting, women are more likely to see the benefits of intermittent fasting without their hormones and reproductive system going into all out panic mode.

While we are on the topic of possible disruptions to the female reproductive system, we will discuss a rather odd side effect that some women may possibly experience from intermittent fasting. The female body contains many unique biological mechanisms that are used specifically to aid in pregnancy and ensure the health of a fetus. Unfortunately, but also incredibly admirable, the female body is designed so that in times of hardship, such as starvation, the fetus will survive no matter the costs to the mother.

When resources and nutrition is running low, a growing fetus can actually cause hormonal changes in the woman's body to reroute vital nutrients to itself. Often times when women are following any sort of fasting protocol, when they break the fast they experience severe, insatiable hunger. This is the female body's way of protecting a potential fetus, regardless if there is one or there's not. Because a woman's body is so uniquely designed to develop and nourish a growing baby, it will actually do whatever it takes to maintain an internal environment conducive to a baby's growth, even if there isn't one there!

To mitigate effects such as this one, experts recommend that women go for several trial fasts before diving headfirst into intermittent fasting. This can be done by consuming all food in an 8-hour feeding window maybe once a week, seeing how your body responds to this, and then adding a day if things go smoothly. However you choose to try out fasting, the key is to be gentle. The last thing you want is to begin an intense fasting regimen and make your body think famine has come and all will be lost if it doesn't protect your growing bundle of joy that isn't actually there. However you choose to begin intermittent fasting, ease into it and the benefits will follow suit.

Another hormonal issue that women need to consider when

beginning intermittent fasting, is their estrogen levels. While the male and female bodies both contain estrogen as well as testosterone, we all know that males contain much more testosterone than women, and women more estrogen than men. These hormones work to provide certain physical and emotional aspects that are unique to the different sexes.

Estrogen, the primary female sex hormone, can actually make it harder or easier for a woman to stick with any dietary plan, especially intermittent fasting. The different craving levels will change depending on certain periods of the menstrual cycle throughout the month. The reason for this is because the hormone estrogen actually decreases appetite by reducing a woman's sensitivity to feeding cues, causing you to feel hungry less often. At certain periods in the menstrual cycle, such as the periovulatory phase, food intake is at its lowest. Likewise, during later periods in the menstrual cycle such as the follicular and luteal phases, food intake is actually increased.

But what does this mean for you? Well, assuming that you plan to adhere to intermittent fasting as a lifestyle, you are likely to have certain periods of the month when it just seems harder to stick to your feeding window. You may think you are just not exercising enough self control, or that you are slacking in your commitment to eating healthier, when really you are just the victim of a hormonal fluctuation that's out of your control. While there is no way to stop the fluctuation of estrogen in your body, (none that you want to try anyway) you can mitigate the intense hunger cravings in the same way that we've talked about reducing or preventing other unwanted side effects. Exercise moderation with intermittent fasting, especially when you first begin this lifestyle. As a female, your body is extremely sensitive to hormonal alterations and is likely to respond adversely if you go from your normal eating routine straight into a prolonged fast.

Although this chapter may seem to have portrayed intermittent fasting in a negative light, the hazards that we have discussed are all easily avoidable. As a woman, your body is designed to protect not only you, but even another human life growing inside of you through the body's delicate hormone balance and biological mechanisms. As long as you approach intermittent fasting from a reasonable perspective with this new found awareness, I truly believe that you can experience the many benefits available from this lifestyle, without falling victim to the possible detriments that are out there.

Remember that moderation is key when starting this protocol. The body is extremely intelligent at sensing small changes or fluctuations in your internal and external environments. The body will turn to drastic measures to protect itself and maintain homeostasis. Therefore, when beginning any sort of new diet or exercise program, you should gradually implement the change into your day-to-day life.

You would never attempt to run a marathon without starting a progressive training program. Maybe running a mile every day until that became easy, and then moving on to running half-marathons, etc. The same logic applies to intermittent fasting. It's not a good idea to go from eating your normal breakfast, lunch, and dinner, then suddenly go 16 hours without eating.

You know when you see those commercials play on television advertising a type of medicine? Then at the end of the ad an unnecessarily fast speaker chimes in to list off about 50 possible side effects listed in the fine print at the bottom of your screen? Although the side effects they mention only occur in a very small percentage of individuals that take the medicine, they still have to inform you of them for your health and safety. This chapter serves to delve into that purpose and thoroughly explain any of the female issues that could possibly arrive, so you are aware of them and know how to avoid them.

Although there are some possible health hazards that can occur for women seeking intermittent fasting as a healthy eating habit, this is only the exception to the rule. If you will follow the advice on how to prevent the side effects that we have discussed, you are more than likely to have a pleasant and beneficial experience as you begin this journey. Even ibuprofen has been known to cause everything from diarrhea to shortness of breath in some people, but I doubt that you consider these side effects every time you get a headache! Rest assured that with careful planning and self awareness, intermittent fasting will help the large majority of women achieve their weight loss and fitness goals.

"To lengthen thy life, lessen thy meals". -Benjamin Franklin

Chapter 4: Having A Healthy Mentality For Intermittent Fasting

In our world today, the standard of beauty and what constitutes the ideal physique has promoted and even praised unrealistic expectations for men and women alike. Everywhere you look there are cover models on magazines with chiseled abs, models fitting perfectly in size zero dresses, actors in every movie with physiques the average person could probably never obtain. Being exposed to this sort of standard from every angle day after day, can most definitely wear on our self-image and confidence.

Like I said, this goes for both men and women, but I think we can all agree that women bear the brunt of this aspect of life. The media does its very best to make you believe that you cannot be considered pretty, or in shape, unless you mimic these unrealistic expectations presented to you in the magazines and television. Sadly, this not only leads to lowered self-esteem in large numbers of women, but sometimes it can escalate into health disorders.

To try and cope with these expectations, some individuals develop a severe eating disorder known as bulimia. This is a disorder where someone consumes usually a large amount of food, feels guilty, and then becomes so worried that it will be detrimental to their physique that they actually induce vomiting, or take a large amount of laxatives, in a desperate attempt to reverse the situation. These methods are usually referred to as "purging." This disorder can wreak absolute havoc on the body. People with bulimia commonly have severe stomach distortion from overeating, electrolyte imbalance from severe dehydration, ulcers covering the lining of their esophagus from the constant stomach acid coming up from vomiting, and tooth decay also due to stomach acid. Although men and women both suffer from this disorder, women are much more prone to it. The United States Department of Health and Human Services reports that as many as 2% of women suffer from this eating disorder.

Another severe eating disorder many people suffer from is anorexia. This results in a person limiting their food intake to dangerously low levels for fear of gaining weight, exercising far too much in an attempt to burn calories. They often have a severely distorted body image in which they feel that their obese, when in reality they are far too thin. Once again, even though this disorder affects both men and women, it is predominately a female condition, with an estimated 1 in 20 women in the United States suffering from anorexia. This disorder also has terrible health implications such as heart problems, anemia, and extremely high-risk pregnancies.

Eating disorders are a real problem, and women are overwhelmingly more prone to developing them. So, how does all of this information relate to intermittent fasting, you may wonder? Well, my point is that with the way intermittent fasting places on emphasis on specific periods of fasting, followed by strict eating windows, it can sometimes cause women to develop an unhealthy obsession with food.

If your body is still getting used to going extended periods of time without eating, there is a greater likelihood that when the feeding window begins you will be so hungry that you overdo it. If you are really wanting to see results from following this protocol and are ashamed of yourself for consuming an excessive amount of food, the guilt you feel might even lead you to becoming bulimic, purging yourself to try and undo the situation. Likewise, if after adhering to intermittent fasting for some time and not seeing the results that you hoped for, you may start to feel like what you are doing is not enough. This can cause women to become more predisposed to developing anorexia.

When this happens, it is easy to see how someone may shorten their eating window far too much, or barely eat any food at all during the allotted feeding time. Although women must be aware and cautious of these eating disorders when beginning intermittent fasting, this becomes even more important if they have any prior history of eating disorders, as the likelihood of relapsing increases substantially. To prevent any of these eating disorders from rearing their ugly head, one needs to make sure that their perspective is in the right place. The first thing you need to remember is that intermittent fasting is about becoming a healthier, happier version of you.

Remember all of the benefits you can enjoy that we discussed earlier? Well these don't mean anything if you develop an extremely unhealthy relationship with food in the process. It is important that you keep in mind why you started it in the first place; to better yourself. The second thing to keep in mind is that you are a human being (shocker right?). We are imperfect creatures with limited self-control, we make mistakes.

I can assure you that if you choose to begin intermittent fasting, there will be times that you make mistakes. Maybe that eating window just cannot wait, and you give in to the hot and ready sign at Krispy Kreme on your way home. Sometimes you may consume a few too many calories when those precious feeding hours begin. In nutrition, fitness, and even life in general, it is never the small, infrequent things that yield long term results. What you need to remember is that the things you do HABITUALLY are what will make or break you.

If you eat a terrible diet routinely and randomly decide to eat healthy for only one day, do you think you are going to immediately lose 10 pounds? Is going to the gym twice a year going to get you in fantastic shape and allow you to reach your fitness goals? Having said that, slipping up on your diet from time to time or missing a workout every once in a while is not going to ruin your weight-loss and exercise goals. Anything worth achieving, especially when it comes to your body, is not going to happen overnight.

However, if you consistently follow the intermittent fasting protocol, or any other diet for that matter, then even with the minor setbacks that happen you are still on the path to your goals! When it comes to intermittent fasting, you need to understand that this is merely a tool at your disposal that you are choosing to use to become a healthier person. You must never let something like this control you, after all, you are the one in control choosing to live this lifestyle, and you have the power to stop or change the rules at any time.

In your journey with intermittent fasting, it is of the utmost importance that you never lose sight of the big picture. Remember that food is not the most important thing in your life, and preoccupation with eating should never get in the way of the things that matter most to you. Although cruel, societal definitions and images portrayed by the media are giving us a horrible definition of what it means to be healthy. Most of the muscular men shown in movies and magazine covers are abusing harmful substances such as anabolic steroids, and a large number of women modeling the latest fashions are secretly suffering from the eating disorders that we discussed.

If you let it, comparing yourself to these people will do nothing but rob you of your joy and discourage you from trying to be your best. The only measuring stick that you should stand next to in your journey should be your former self. It is amazing how much fitness and nutrition mirror all of life itself. In everything you do, you should wake up every morning trying to improve yourself from the you that fell asleep last night. Never let anyone tell you that you are not good enough and that you're not capable of reaching your health and wellness goals. You are more than capable of achieving them with the right amount of knowledge and commitment.

Intermittent fasting is a tried and true method of eating that human beings have been utilizing for thousands and thousands of years, without even really knowing the true extent of its benefits. When it comes to women's health and wellness, always remember that YOU are in control of your life. Modern media's definition of what you should look like and how you should eat are in your face everywhere you turn in your daily life. It is time to change the way that our society defines healthy eating and what it means to have an ideal physique. Do not let anyone or anything define who you are and what you can accomplish.

Chapter 5: Getting Started With Intermittent Fasting And How To Do The Different Fasting Methods

Now that we have discussed what intermittent fasting entails, as well as the precautions that women following this eating pattern should take, I believe you are ready to begin this journey. To begin this chapter we will start off by getting you prepared to begin intermittent fasting effectively. There are actually several different styles of intermittent fasting, and we will break down each of these techniques and point out some of their unique benefits. Although any approach to fasting must follow some basic foundational steps, there are minor tweaks for each method. After completing this chapter, feel free to choose any of the methods listed and go from there!

The first thing you need to do to get ready to begin intermittent fasting, or any other diet plan for that matter, is to consult your doctor. Make sure that this lifestyle is not going to harm you due to any underlying health conditions you may have. The health hazards that we discussed in chapter two are avoidable, but there are in fact some people who should probably not begin intermittent fasting. For example, people suffering from diabetes will most likely receive more harm than good from this lifestyle due to their already unstable blood sugar levels. Your doctor will be able to give you the go ahead on this eating style and advise you of any further precautions you should take to make sure you remain healthy for the duration.

The next step to take is to make sure that you are really committed to giving this lifestyle a chance. This is going to be a pretty big change in your day-to-day schedule, and may not be the easiest thing to stick with at the beginning. Keep in mind that your daily fasting periods are going to seem difficult to begin with. Not only will your body be surprised and wondering what exactly is going on, but you will be tempted at every angle to stray from your plan. Don't worry, this is natural. Old habitual temptations always happen when you bring about a healthy new change in your life.

Those morning donuts in the break room at work will probably seem more delicious than usual, and when your friends invite you out to your favorite frozen yogurt stand after work, they may not understand why you choose not to go all of the sudden. Remember, this is your journey, and you cannot expect everyone in your life to understand it. Before you even consider starting intermittent fasting, make sure you are in the right place mentally so that you can stick with it long enough to make a fair assessment as to whether or not this is right for you.

Once your doctor gives you the green light and you are mentally prepared for intermittent fasting, give it a little trial run for a while. Start off with one day of fasting per week, whether that is an entire day or having a set eating/fasting window. When you are comfortable with this day of fasting and feel like you can stick with it, then you can progress to a more regular fasting schedule such as the ones I will now explain below.

The first method of intermittent fasting that we will breakdown is commonly referred to as the Lean gains method. This protocol was made popular by Martain Berkhan, and is one of the more popular fasting options. The Lean gains method, for women, breaks down each day into a 14 hour fast, followed by a 10 hour eating window. While in the fasting period, you are to eat no calories whatsoever. Always drink water, and feel free to consume other things such as black coffee with calorie free sweeteners, sugar free gum, or even diet soda in moderation.

The majority of followers of the Lean gains method prefer to make their fast last throughout the night, therefore they are only abstaining from food a short period of time while they are actually awake. For example, if you go to bed at 10 o'clock and wake up at 6, you have already completed 8 hours of your fast. This method stresses the importance of maintaining a consistent eating window to ensure your hormonal levels do not fluctuate too drastically.

Another aspect of the Lean gains program, is that it dictates what makes up the majority of your diet on days you workout versus rest days. On you workout days, you should get the majority of your calories from carbohydrates instead of fat. When you work out, your body is going to require more energy and the most readily available form comes from consuming carbs. On rest days, this method recommends getting more calories from fat instead of carbohydrates. Another important point to mention is that your protein intake should remain relatively stable every day, and by stable I mean fairly high. Remember that no matter where you are getting your calories from (carbohydrates, fat, protein), you should be consuming whole unprocessed foods. These can consists of fruits, vegetables, lean meats, and nuts.

Many people enjoy the Lean gains protocol because eating times are not strictly specified as long as they occur during your ten-hour window. Most people that follow this method will tell you that if you consume three meals during feeding time, then being consistent with the plan will seem easier, because we are already programmed to consume three meals a day anyway (breakfast, lunch, dinner). While certainly effective, some people find the caloric specificity on workout versus rest days difficult to stick with.

To someone without much prior knowledge of what food groups contain lots of carbs, fat, and/or protein, this process may seem confusing and hard to maintain. However, with a little bit of research and practice, you will establish a better understanding of what foods to choose when you need certain macronutrients. All in all, the Lean gains method of intermittent fasting is a fairly simple, effective style to begin with and will yield great results if you stick with it.

Another popular method of intermittent fasting is the eat stop eat program made popular by Brad Pilon. In this program, you simply fast for an entire 24-hour day, once or twice per week. On the non-fasting days, you just follow your usual eating patterns with no regards to fasting. As with most styles of intermittent fasting, you are only required to not consume any calories during the fast, things such as coffee, water, and diet soda are permitted.

The main explanation for this method of fasting is that you are reducing your weekly caloric intake, while still being able to enjoy your favorite foods. However, you still have to make intelligent food choices on non-fasting days. Sure, two days without fasting per week will cut down on calories and yield many of the benefits we discussed in chapter two, but if you chow down on fried Oreos and French fries all day the rest of the week, you are going nowhere (I assume this need not be explained).

The biggest convenience of the eat stop eat program is its flexibility. Starting off, going an entire 24 hours without food may be too difficult, so feel free to pick a couple days per week and go as long as you can without eating on those days with the end goal of 24 hours in mind. This goes back to staying safe as a woman beginning intermittent fasting. Your hormonal levels are already in a delicate balance and not eating for an entire day from the start, may leave you susceptible to health hazards discussed in chapter 3. So make sure you're gentle with yourself and take things one step at a time.

Another great thing about this style of intermittent fasting is that there are no specific foods you must consume, no counting calories, weighing meals, or anything like that. As long as you don't turn your eating days into a contest between you and your stomach, and remain sensible, you can reap the benefits of this plan without making huge changes to your everyday life. The cons of the eat stop eat method are understandable, but really come down to a lack of self-control. Some people report that after their 24 hour fast is over, they are far more prone to binge and overdo it when it comes time to eat. If you suffer from a lack of self-control, this plan may not be a perfect fit for you.

The next popular form of intermittent fasting is called the warrior diet, created and promoted by Ori Hofmekler. The warrior diet is one of the more strict forms of intermittent fasting and may not be for everyone, but it does promote some interesting benefits. Basically, this diet instructs you to fast for 20 hours a day, eating one large meal at night.

Hofmekler explains that humans are naturally designed to be nocturnal eaters, and a large evening meal aligns with our natural circadian rhythm. A unique aspect of the warrior diet is that the fasting period is actually not a fast by definition, as you are allowed to eat things such as raw fruits and vegetables, freshly squeezed juice, and small servings of protein.

This is apparently supposed to boost your sympathetic nervous system, which is what you have probably heard referred to as the body's "fight or flight" response. If the sympathetic nervous system is engaged throughout the day, you can expect to experience more alertness and energy, while also promoting fat burning. The other side of the nervous system, the parasympathetic nervous system, is commonly referred to as the "rest and digest" response. With the four-hour eating window at the end of each day, the warrior diet is supposed to promote relaxation and repair of the body through the large meal you consume.

To further emphasize the strict guidelines of this diet, even what you eat is specified during the eating window. The warrior diet advises you to start your eating window with vegetables, protein, and healthy fats. If you want to eat any more after that, then you are allowed to consume carbohydrates. Followers of this method explain that being allowed a few snacks here and there during the day makes the warrior diet easier to stick with. The cons of this method are pretty obvious with this one; many people find the strict guidelines difficult to fit into their lifestyle on a regular basis. The warrior diet is one of the more interesting forms of intermittent fasting, if you are ready to flex your self-control muscle and alter your way of life fairly significantly, this method may be right for you!

If all of the methods of intermittent fasting sound interesting for you, you don't actually have to choose just one. The fat loss forever program, created by John Romaniello and Dan Go, actually incorporates aspects of several other methods of intermittent fasting into one program. The basics of the fat loss forever program go as follows: you get one cheat day per week where any food is allowed, any time of the day (within sensible guidelines).

After this cheat day you go on a 36 hour fast where you consume nothing but calorie free sustenance such as coffee, diet soda, water, etc. Once this fast comes to an end, the rest of the week alternates from one intermittent fasting protocol to another, until you come full circle back to the original cheat day. While a 36-hour fast does sound tedious, the creators of the fat loss forever program advise you to select your busiest days to be the fasting period, that way your mind is engaged on something other than your hunger.

This is a pretty complex fasting program, but it also features a daily calendar breaking down exactly how you are supposed to eat each day of the week. Fat loss forever gets praise for keeping intermittent fasting fresh. Instead of following the exact same fasting and eating schedule every day, you are constantly in a dynamic cycle that will keep you from getting bored with it. People also love the full cheat day that comes with this method. If you struggle with handling cheat days sensibly or maintaining structure in your life, this program may not be the best way for you to approach intermittent fasting.

The last popular method of intermittent fasting that we will discuss was created by Dr. James Johnson and is called alternate-day fasting. This is a really simple form of fasting that involves eating very few calories one day, and eating normal the next. More specifically with the low-calorie day, Dr.Johnson suggests taking your normal daily caloric intake and dividing that number by 5. For example, if you usually consume 2,500 calories per day, shoot for around 500 calories on your low-calorie days.

To make starting this method as smooth as possible, you are advised to get your calories on the low-calorie days from meal replacement shakes. This allows you to sip on them throughout the day, instead of only getting to eat a few tiny meals. However, you are only supposed to do this on the first two weeks of beginning alternate-day fasting, whereas after this you need to be getting your calories from real foods. People who have tried this method of intermittent fasting report remarkable weight loss success, the biggest benefit of this program. As with other protocols, if you are prone to binging on cheat days, you may find that on days you are allowed to eat normal, you overdo it big time.

These are the five most popular methods of intermittent fasting.

While they vary slightly with different rules and guidelines, you really can't go wrong either way. As I mentioned in the beginning of this book, the best diet is the one that you will stick with. Pick a method of fasting and try it out. If it seems to be something that you can manage, by all means stick with it. If not, then you can try another form of intermittent fasting out until you find what works for you! Whatever plan you decide on, always keep your health and safety first and foremost. As a woman pursuing the intermittent fasting lifestyle, always practice moderation, easing into the method, and making sure you maintain a healthy relationship with food!

"I fast for greater physical and mental efficiency." -Plato

Conclusion

Thank you so very much for taking the time to read this book. I sincerely hope you are now equipped with a solid understanding of exactly what intermittent fasting is. Just as importantly, it is my wish that you are aware of the safe way for a woman to go about getting started with this lifestyle. There are a wide variety of methods that you can utilize on your fasting journey, the end goal is that all of them lead to the same destination: a healthier and happier you!

Remember that you are in control of your nutrition, health, and overall wellness. You do not have to follow intermittent fasting to achieve your goals, but this lifestyle is certainly a valuable tool to assist you with the health and physique you are striving for. Always remember that you are the one in control of what you eat and when you eat. If you choose to use intermittent fasting, that is a conscious choice that you are in complete control over. Never let any diet or exercise regimen gain control of you.

Intermittent fasting, although not a new idea by any means, has reemerged into the spotlight of the health and fitness industry and is now becoming the go-to nutrition plan for many people. If you sincerely commit to taking action and you try out this lifestyle for yourself, then it might just be the exact tool you needed to reach the health and weight goals that you desire. Now you have gained the understanding of how the female body works with intermittent fasting, and the knowledge of what to do, the choice is yours!

Finally, if you enjoyed this book, it would be greatly appreciated if you could share your thoughts and leave an Amazon review for me!

Thank you and good luck!